I0146151

AN A-Z

OF YOU!

Helping your amazing
body to last a
lifetime

Karlene Rickard

Filament Publishing

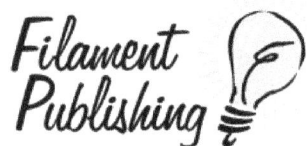

Published by
Filament Publishing Ltd
16, Croydon Road,
Beddington, Croydon CR0 4PA
www.filamentpublishing.com
+44(0) 208 688 2598

The A-Z of You by Karlene Rickard

ISBN 978-1-912256-38-9

© Karlene Rickard 2017

The right of Karlene Rickard to be identified as the author
of this work has been asserted by her in accordance with
the Designs and Copyrights Act 1988

All rights reserved
No part of this work may be copied in any
way without the prior written permission
of the publishers

Printed IngramSpark

DEDICATION

I would like to dedicate this book to my son, Pianki, my granddaughter Maitlyn a very good friend Jim Sullivan of Thoughts for Others who supported me in so many ways and all those who are searching for their purpose in life.

The information in this book comes from my studies as a science teacher, life experiences, books and my research.

ACKNOWLEDGEMENTS

Firstly I have to give God thanks for the inspiration, revelation and instruction for this book, through a Deacon I met in Jamaica. Then to Ankhara and Donna who have edited, proof read and given useful feedback also, Margaret Robinson who sacrificed many days to be a sounding board, made useful suggestions and carried out the overall edition and proof read. I would also thank those who tolerated me and also thank Chris for sound advice and his expertise in formatting, laying out and designing this book.

Thanks to Jeffrey Plaffkow Optician of Optical World for all of his help.

Foreword

The A-Z Of You is an amazing piece of work by Ms. Karlene Rickard.

Ms. Rickard incorporates her knowledge of God's creation and her scientific background to produce an interesting read that informs you of the extraordinary working of the human body.

This book will expose you to parts of your body you may not have known about, or perhaps overlooked, giving you a newfound appreciation of what you already have. Your body is the most advanced computer system ever created; if treated appropriately will last you a lifetime and allow you to enjoy your life to the fullest.

A-Z Of You I believe exposes you to the genius Creator and how as human beings we have within us the same DNA that enables us to be creators on earth.

Iroro Agba.

ORGANS OF THE
HUMAN BODY

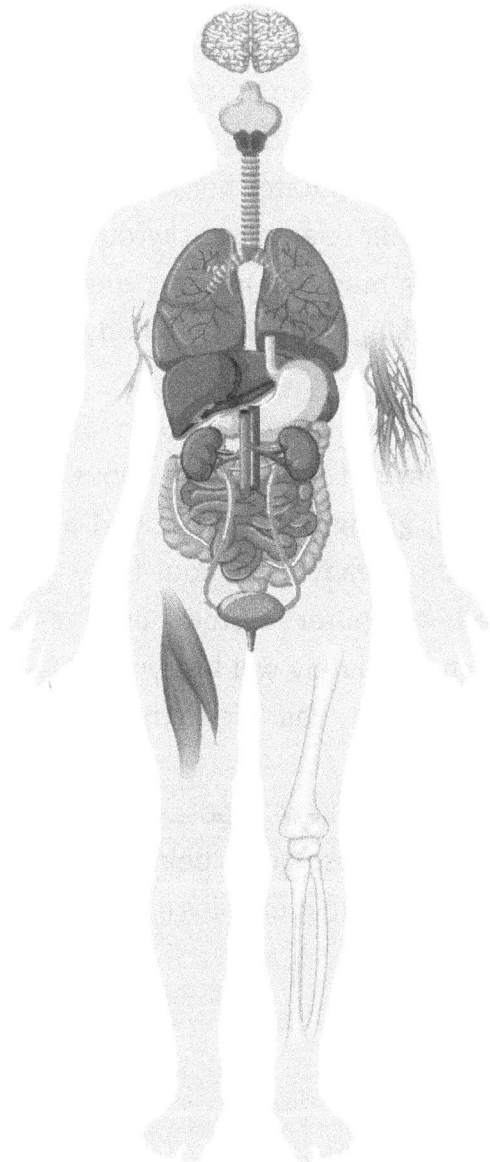

INTRODUCTION

This might come as a surprise to you but the body which we complain so much about - "I" am too fat," - "I am too thin," "My joints ache" is truly phenomenal. As a matter of fact the Word of God says we are fearfully and wonderfully made. What I am saying is, if you were to understand and appreciate the real person you are, and the complexity of your body functions, you would probably be shocked.

I embarked on this journey to provide non biologist with an insight into the incredible workings of the human being, the function of some parts you have never thought or heard about. The body is made up of visible organs like the skin, hidden organs like the heart. The organs are made up of cells; inside the cells there are structures known as organelles one example is mitochondrion.

My intention is to make this information accessible by drawing on the many parallels of body parts between machines and human systems.

This book combines my fascination with the human body and my love of photography and filming. One day while filming I took a strong interest in the mechanics of the camera.

I became intrigued with its similarity to the human eye. This engaged my interest in the relationship between other body parts, with various inventions and systems developed by man. I then concluded that the body in essence has provided a blue print for many everyday objects, structures and systems created by man. There is nothing new in this world; all that is without is within. However unlike man, God has no copyright and graciously offers us the right to respectfully copy all of his creation.

Over the years my inspiration became more profound. During my vacation in Jamaica in November to December 2016, on my last Sunday I attended Duhaney New Testament Church of God in Kingston. Solomon Wisdom prayed for me and revealed that there is a special book within me. I was quite elated. The Thursday of that week on my way to the Bath Fountain Hot Spring Spa in St Thomas, which is a yearly practice, it is therapy for the Multiple Sclerosis, (MS) with which I have been diagnosed. While enroute I believe God began revealing this A to Z to me. I was so excited that after the revelation of each letter I screamed.

Having written three of my previous books in an A-Z format I decided to carry through the same practise with this book. However, this A to Z is not definitive; you may have your own A to Z or you could even be inspired to make a machine or develop a mechanical system.

The human body is a unique structure. Under careful scrutiny you would be astounded at the surreal relationships of different machines, organisations, systems and human body parts.

Furthermore, I would like to encourage readers to appreciate their bodies and the bodies of other people, especially parents who are nurturing young children. The effective function of the body depends on some hidden parts known as organelles. This book shows the parallel between various parts of the human body, both visible and invisible/hidden.

After the masseur treated me I went and sat in the hot spring which I had never done in all the twenty years I had actually visited the site. In the pool I was actually dancing and thanking God whilst oblivious to the fact that one of my my legs was getting burnt; I had felt nothing. When I got out of the spring, a lady exclaimed, "The skin is falling from your leg." I looked down at my legs and I was stunned. The skin was indeed falling from my right ankle; this resulted in me suffering severe burns. The therapist unwittingly rubbed it with pimento oil which compounded the situation.

On my return to the UK I was immediately admitted to hospital. They transferred me to the special hospital where I was given a skin graft and antibiotics for the infection which resulted from the oil.

In this book I have listed my A to Z of those body parts and linked them with structural or operational machines or systems in the everyday world.

I hope this text will inspire everyone to be more discerning. You could become the next inventor or developer of an idea or actualize your true destiny instead of competing with others for what is not actually your calling.

I believe many of the illnesses we experience are unconsciously self-inflicted due to unawareness and lack of knowledge; therefore we often fail to maintain our bodies appropriately. A case in point, in 1982 I was totally paralysed; six years later after numerous tests I was diagnosed with Remitting and Relapsing Multiple Sclerosis. My first experience with medication caused hallucination and there was a possibility of experiencing fits. I abandoned the medication after I had a daily revelation on how to manage the condition which I obeyed. Every part listed in this book with the exception of the penis and the zygote were highlighted and carefully revealed. By faith I obeyed and employed the appropriate natural means to care for them.

Today thirty-five years later I am mobile supported by a rollator or a walking stick, I can manage my personal care, social and dietary needs. Currently I serve as a Bereavement

Voluntary counsellor in a large hospital in the UK, an International Trainer of Parent Facilitators and a Motivational Speaker.

For each exterior body part, organ or organelle listed in this A to Z I have challenged you to ensure you are not under-nourishing or abusing them.

Karlene

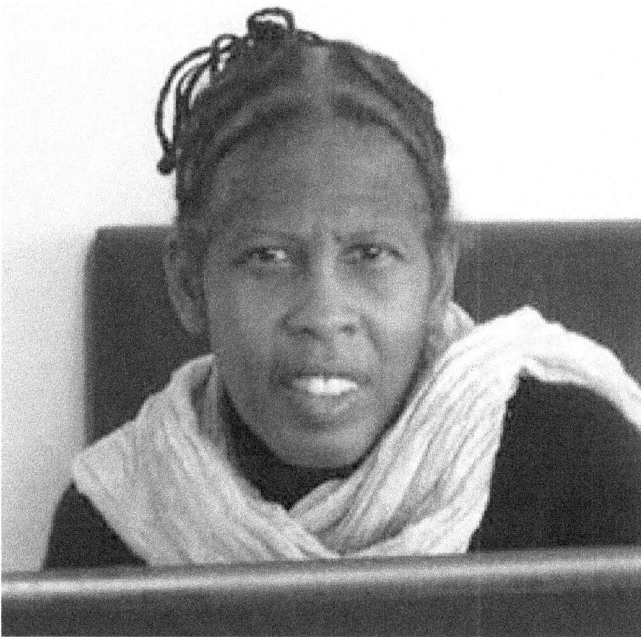

"Everything that is within is without"

•Basic Neuron Types•

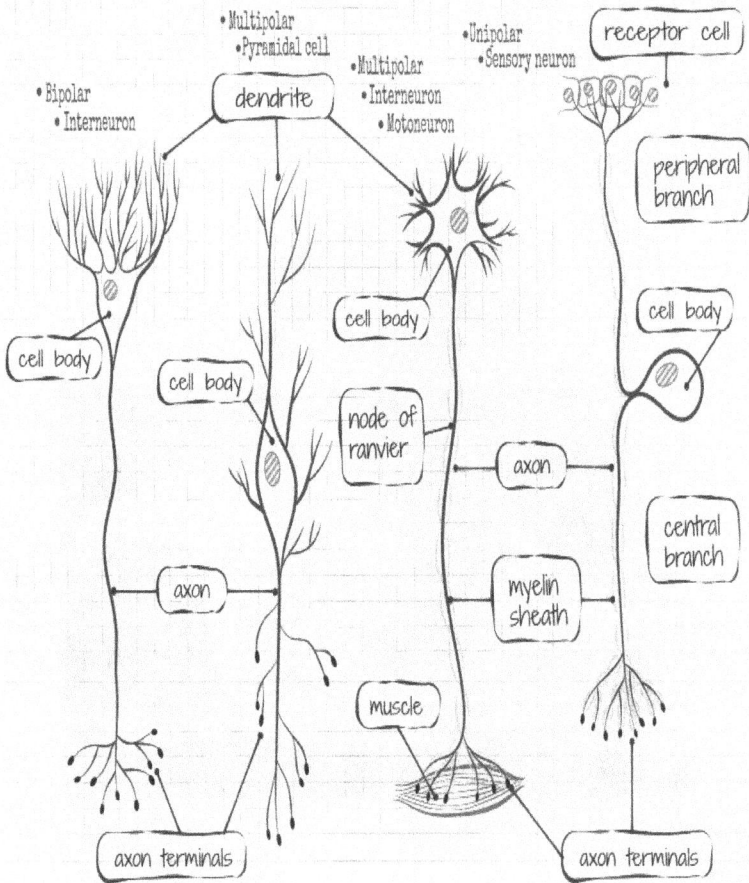

- Multipolar
  - Pyramidal cell

- Multipolar
  - Interneuron
  - Motoneuron

- Unipolar
  - Sensory neuron

- Bipolar
  - Interneuron

receptor cell

dendrite

peripheral branch

cell body

cell body

cell body

cell body

node of ranvier

axon

central branch

axon

myelin sheath

muscle

axon terminals

axon terminals

The A TO Z of YOU!

Before we begin our consideration of how the Human Bodies prallel parts and parallel systems of the modern world, we will begin with the Axon. This is one of the most important basic structures of the Human Body and it begins with A.

A -Axon / Electrical cable

AXON, This is an invisible structural, part of the neuron which makes up the nervous system. Messages travel from outside and inside our bodies every waking moment. The axon can be damaged through brain injuries. It is paramount to wear helmets in related activities thus protecting the head from blows.

An axon is a long, slender projection of the parts of the nerve cell or neuron (Axon, cell body and dendrites). The axons are covered by a protein structure known as the myelin sheath. The axon transmits information through electrical impulse to different muscles and glands. If the myelin sheath is damaged, exposing the fibres which are known as scarring; it prevents the electrical impulses from travelling along the axon.

An axon generates a single electrical impulse called a spike which travels down the axon to activate its synapses| (structures at the end of nerves and deliver tiny chemicals of neurotransmitter to its neighbours. These spikes are all-or-nothing, (they don't reverse) similar to binary ones and zeros in a computer. The structure conducts electrical impulses away from one area of the body that receives it, to the area necessary for response. An example: if one's leg was trapped, this would stimulate the axon to carry impulse from the leg to the brain which would inform the muscles to correct the situation.

The Electric Cable is structured and functions like an Axon. Like the Axon an electric cable is a main wire which contains two or more wires running side by side, together, to form a single assembly. Each electric wire is covered with a plastic covering, like the neuron covered with the myelin sheath, to prevent the naked wires from touching each other. This is to prevent short-circuiting which will prevent the electricity current from flowing to the electric appliance from the source of the electric current through the electric socket. The message is transmitted through electric impulses.

B –BRAIN/COMPUTER

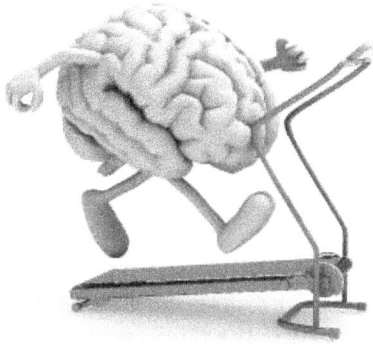

BRAIN

The brain is a very sensitive organ. It's an essential organ for healthy mental and physical well-being. It is stimulated by social and mental activities. In order to generate and maintain the health of the brain, a regular diet is necessary: fish, vegetables, high levels of Vitamin C and antioxidants to inhibit free radicals which kill the healthy cells. It is paramount to stay mentally active and keep the brain healthy and work through our emotional issues so that we will be able to be emotionally stable. We should never stop learning; we ought to try taking a different route to work from time to time, or brush your teeth with the hand we don't normally use. We ought to read more regularly and challenge ourselves with our reading selection.

For basic brain stimulation, we should try to solve puzzles and play games of strategy. We could also learn to play a musical instrument.

The brain has around 100 billion nerve cells. It also has 1,000 billion other cells, which cover the nerve cells and the parts of the nerve cells which form the links between one cell and another, feeding them and keeping them healthy.

The brain keeps on growing until you are about 20 years old. By then the brain has made lots of links which it no longer needs so it is able to shed any unwanted connections and still have billions of brain cells left to cope with whatever you may want to do. The brain can still make new connections even when one is 100 years old. The left side of the brain is analytical, usually better at problem solving, maths and writing.

The right side of the brain is creative and helps you to be good at art or music.

The brain stores all sorts of information in the memory, including facts and figures and all the smells, tastes and things you have seen, heard or touched. The brain can also find and retrieve things that you have remembered.

The adult brain weighs about 1.5kg. Your brain is protected inside your skull and is cushioned by cerebral-spinal fluid but it could still be damaged if it is hit or bumps into something hard.

The computer, like the brain, does its primary work in a part of the machine we cannot see, a control centre that converts data input to information output. This control centre, called the Central Processing Unit (CPU), is a highly complex, extensive set of electronic circuitry that executes stored program instructions. All computers, large and small, must have a central processing unit. The central processing unit consists of two parts: The Control Unit and The Arithmetic/logic Unit. Each part has a specific function.

The data storage has a relationship to the central processing unit. Computers use two types of storage: Primary storage and Secondary storage. The CPU interacts closely with primary storage, or main memory, referring to it for both instructions and data.

The computer's memory holds data only temporarily, at the time the computer is executing a programme. Secondary storage holds permanent or semi-permanent data on some external magnetic or optical medium. The diskettes and CD-ROM discs that you have seen with personal computers are secondary storage devices, as are hard disc devices.

The computer, like the brain, processes and recalls information from memory and computes information; both have circuitries and use electrical impulses. They both operate as enclosed invisible operation systems.

C - CIRCULATORY SYSTEM/ TRANSPORTATION SYSTEM

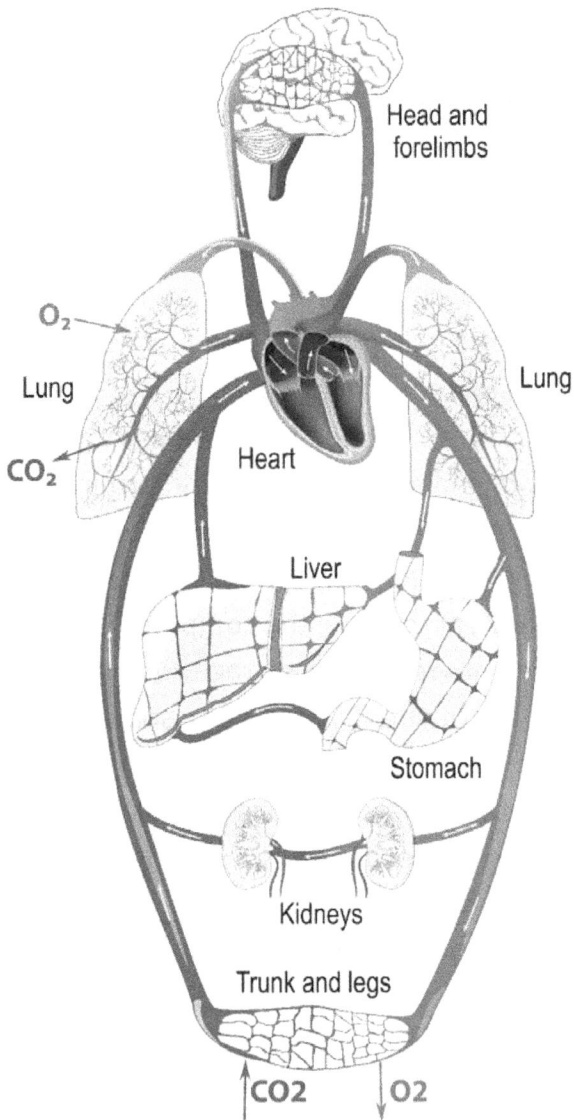

Head and forelimbs

O_2

Lung

CO_2

Lung

Heart

Liver

Stomach

Kidneys

Trunk and legs

$CO2$ $O2$

To keep the circulatory system healthy, it is important to exercise on a regular basis. This format includes excercise like: walking, jogging, running, biking, skating, jumping and swimming. All are excellent for developing a strong cardiovascular system. When running be careful not to run on the streets and put too much stress on your knees. Run in parks where possible. Massage stimulates many of the body's organs and stimulates blood flow. We should ensure we eat a healthy diet and avoid smoking. Avoid junk and oily foods.

The body's circulatory system is made up of blood vessels. The main artery is known as the aorta but there are smaller vessels called veins, arteries and very small vessels called the capillaries. In the vessels, blood which is water, red and white cells carry food, nutrients, chemicals around the body to different organs and take waste materials from organs and discharge them from the body through systems of excretion.

The transport system is made up of large main roads known as motor-ways or high ways rather like the aorta and lesser roads known as A and B roads rather like the veins and arteries, then tracks similar to the capillaries. As the blood flows through the veins, arteries and capillaries picking up and delivering a range of substances, the transport is a route for lorries, trucks and various vehicles on which people and goods are carried from one place to another. The veins and arteries carry things in one direction like the one way road in our transportation system.

D –DENDRITES / WIFI

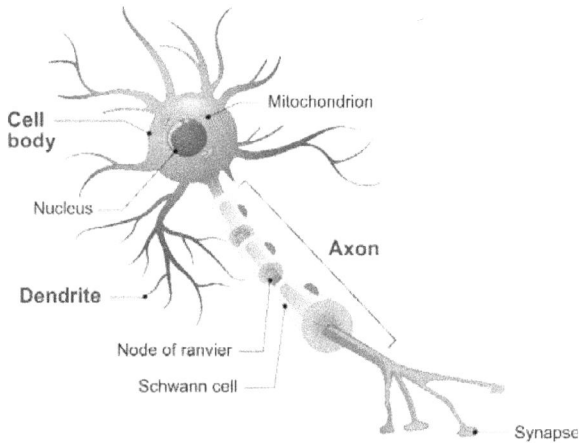

To keep the dendrites healthy, avoid negative and toxic thoughts and being judgemental. These processes produce toxic chemicals which destroy the communication system between the dendrites around the body.

Dendrites are treelike extensions at the beginning of a neuron (nerve cell) that help increase the surface area of the cell body. These tiny protrusions receive information from other neurons and transmit electrical stimulation to the cell body.

Neurons (nerve cells) have many dendrites. Some neurons have very small, short dendrites, while other cells possess very long ones. The neurons of the central nervous systems have very long and complex dendrites which then receive signals from as many as a thousand other neurons.

However, some neurons may have only one dendrite, many are short and highly branched. They transmit information to the cell body. These dendrites then receive chemical signals from other neurons, which are then converted into electrical impulses that are transmitted toward the cell body.

If the electrical impulses transmitted inward toward the cell body are large enough, they will generate an action potential. This results in the signal being transmitted down the axon.

The Internet and Wi-Fi systems work in a similar fashion to the Dendrites where wireless messages are sent or received globally. Similarly messages are transmitted to various parts of the body just as cordless messages are sent around the world.

The Internet is (the network of interconnected computers) and communication systems including email, VoIP (Internet telephony, such as Skype), IPTV (television), and P2P file-sharing applications.. The Internet is like a compilation of hundreds of computers (including computing devices such as cell phones and all kinds of automated machines that communicate over the Net). The Web is hundreds of millions of websites, most of which contain links to other pages on the same site and other websites entirely.

If you send an email or browse a webpage, packets of data travel over something like six to ten links between your computer (a browser or client) and the distant computer you're communicating with at the other end (a server). That gives you some idea of how many "layers" of networks are involved in linking any two points on the Internet; there isn't simply a one-to-one connection (at least, not in most).

E -EYE /THE CAMERA

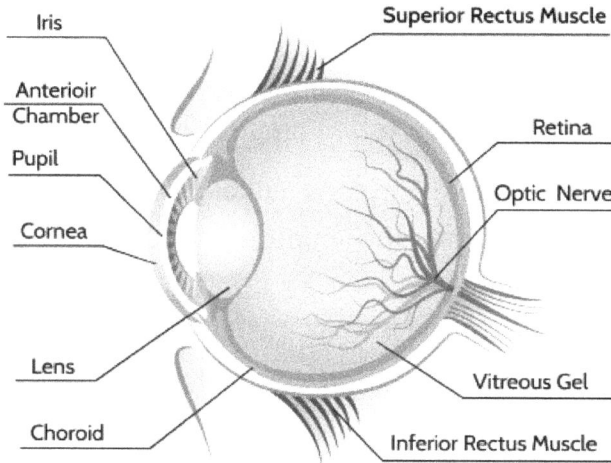

The eye is extremely sensitive. You need to eat lots of green leafy vegetables like spinach, collard and kale which help to avoid muscular degeneration.

It is imperative for us to take vitamins made specifically for eye health. These include: Vitamins A, C, E and B2 and the minerals zinc and selenium. Keep your eyes hydrated. (A simple saline solution can help to lubricate and soothe eyes).

Eat apricots and blueberries, both of which promote good vision. Get plenty of Omega 3 fish oil. It helps clear eyesight and promotes health.

Avoid too much ultra violet rays. Give your eyes a break. If you work at a computer, remember the 20/20/20 rule. Take a break every 20 minutes. For 20 seconds, look at something 20 feet away or farther. This allows your eyes to refocus and relax and prevents the blurry vision that can occur by staring at a computer screen for too long.

The human eye is able to photo shoot instantaneously the minutest detail in a split second.

The human eye sees an object, focuses on it and transmits light through a lens to create an image at the back of the eye. In order to see, we must have light. Light enters the eye through the cornea, the clear front surface of the eye. The light with the image goes to the back of the eye where it lands on the retina which has light sensitive cells, rods for black and white cones for colour. The eye is to convert light into electrochemical impulses that the brain can interpret as visual images.

The various parts of the eye perform different functions that contribute to this purpose like a camera.. The pupil is like the aperture, iris is like a shutter, lens similar, light sensitive cells like film, when the image approaches the camera it is diminished, inverted. The eye has ciliary muscles which stretch or slacken the suspensory ligaments to adjust the shape of the lens.

The iris adjusts the amount of light entering the eye through the pupil. The retina detects light and converts it into electrical impulses which are sent to the brain.

The eye is made up of three coats, enclosing three transparent structures. The outermost layer, known as the fibrous tunic, is composed of the cornea and sclera. The middle layer, known as the vascular tunic, consists of the choroid, ciliary body, and iris.

When you want to take a photograph with a film camera, the light from the image approaches the camera. As you press a button this operates a mechanism called the shutter, which makes a hole (the aperture) open briefly at the front of the camera, allowing light to enter through the lens (a thick piece of glass or plastic mounted on the front). The prism turns the image the right way round. There is a mechanism to focus light onto the photosensitive surface at the back of the camera.

The photosensitive surface detects and records the light which is focused onto it. This can be on photographic film, but digital cameras use a Charge Coupled Device (CCD) which convert light into electrical signals which can be stored. This device allows the user to adjust the focus for nearer or more distant objects.

Aperture allows the user to adjust the amount of light entering the camera in different light conditions. The shutter allows the user to adjust the length of time that light enters the camera, which controls the amount of light to which the photosensitive surface is exposed.

The key difference between a camera and the eye is that a camera does not focus light onto the photosensitive surface by adjusting the shape of the lens. Instead, the focusing screws of the camera move the lens forwards or backwards in order to focus the image onto the photosensitive surface. Like the eye, the image produced by a camera is diminished, inverted and real.

F - FINGERS /GRABBER

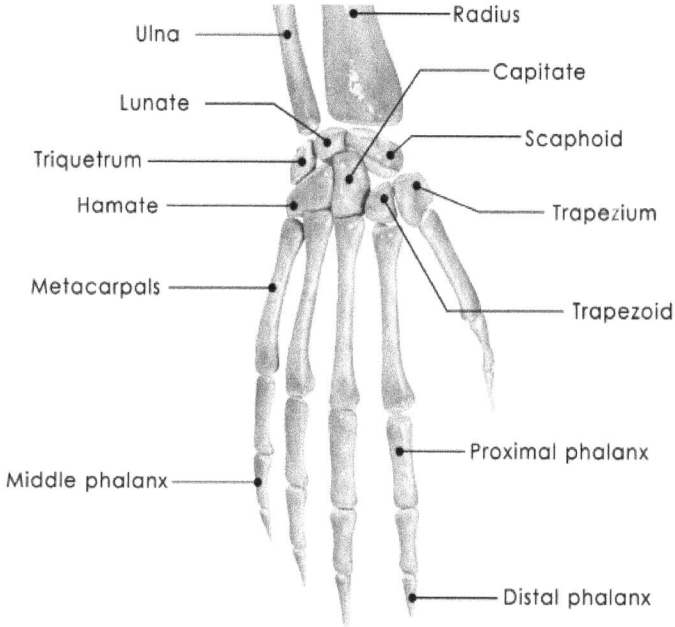

Ulna — Radius

Capitate

Lunate

Scaphoid

Triquetrum

Hamate — Trapezium

Metacarpals

Trapezoid

Proximal phalanx

Middle phalanx

Distal phalanx

It is important that we use the right products to wash and moisturise our hands to ensure the skin doesn't get dry and cracked. It's also important to protect your hands from things that can irritate them, such as the sun, water, and household chores. Regularly cleaning and trimming the finger nails will support growth of strong, healthy nails. Fingers are used to pick up various things especially very small items; the tips grip and then enclose the object.

The technique used depends on whether the object is very large and very heavy, and what sort of shape it has and how easy it is to handle. The long flexor tendons pull the fingers and the thumb together so that they can tightly close around the object. This grip is made possible by the four other fingers flexing and more importantly, the ability of the thumb to be positioned opposite the fingers. With the hand in this position, larger objects such as a stone or a heavy bottle can be held and moved in a controlled way. The greater the weight and the smoother the surface is, the more strength is needed for holding and moving the object. The precision grip is important for delicately handling and moving an object, for example when writing, sewing or drawing. When using the precision grip, the thumb and the index finger work like forceps. The thumb is opposite one or more fingertips, allowing the hand a controlled grip of even very small objects like a pencil or fine instruments. Depending on the weight of the object and the direction and speed of the movement, the brain directs the use of force and coordinates the muscles of the hand.

The Grabber is a small hand held device that is used for picking up small objects.

It consists of a fixed claw finger that is attached to the end of the rod, and another hinged claw finger which is on a spring hinge that causes the claw to fully open when no force is applied.

The sprung finger is attached to the trigger by a length of cord of some kind, which is naturally relaxed and pulled taut by the trigger. At the other end it is attached to the hinged claw. The cord runs down to the claw inside the rod and wraps around the hinged point of the finger starting from the side that is beyond the hinge away from the end of the claw. It then wraps into the inside of the claw on that finger, such that when the cord is pulled taut, the pickers claw is pulled closed, when you release the trigger the sprung hinge pulls against the cord returning the claw to open and the trigger to its unpressed position.

The power grip is better suited for large, heavy objects, and the precision grip is used for small, lighter objects. The power grip is also used for carrying heavy bags or for holding on to a handle, for example. In the power grip, the object is held in the palm of the hand.

G- GUMS/PUTTY

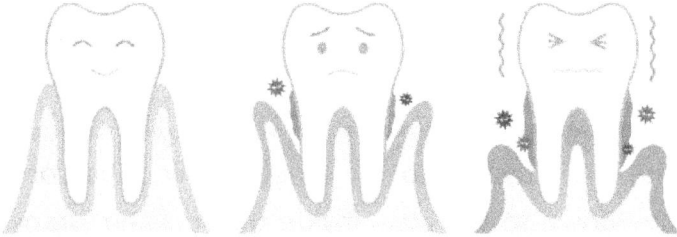

Gingivae (gums) are soft tissues that immediately surround the teeth and bone. Gums protect the bone and the roots of the teeth and The gums keep the teeth intact.

Putty is a soft material that is used to secure glass in a window frame in the same way as the gum is used to protect the edge of glass and keep it secure to the window frame. The difference is that the putty hardens but the gum remains soft.

H –HEART/PUMP

It is essential for your heart to be carefully maintained. Carrying excess weight puts a great deal of strain on the heart. Ensure that you manage your weight by having a healthy, balanced diet. This should be low in fat and sugar, with plenty of fruit and vegetables, combined with regular physical activity.

Eating too many foods that are high in saturated fat can raise the level of cholesterol in our blood. Choose leaner cuts of meat and lower-fat dairy products like 1% fat milk, over full-fat (or whole) milk.

Eat Omega-3 fats which can help protect against heart disease and at least five portions of of fruit and vegetables a day.

Avoid using salt at the table and try adding less to your cooking. Eat fish at least twice a week, including a portion of oily fish. Fish such as mackerel, sardine, fresh tuna and salmon are sources of Omega-3 fats, which can help protect against heart disease.

Pregnant or breastfeeding women shouldn't have more than two portions of oily fish a week.

The human heart is an organ that pumps blood throughout the body via the circulatory system, supplying oxygen and nutrients to the tissues and removing carbon dioxide and other wastes.

The heart is a specialised muscle that contracts regularly and continuously, pumping blood to the body and the lungs. The pumping action is caused by a flow of electricity through the heart that repeats itself in a cycle. If this electrical activity is disrupted – for example by a disturbance in the heart's rhythm known as an 'arrhythmia' – it can affect the heart's ability to pump properly.

The heart's natural pacemaker – the Sinartel (SA) node one of the major elements in the cardiac connection system sends out regular electrical impulses from the top chamber of the heart (the atrium) causing it to contract and pump blood into the bottom chamber (the ventricle). The electrical impulse is then conducted to the ventricles through a form of 'junction box' called the AV node Atrioventular (VS). The electrical node relay station between upper and lower chambers of the heart ensures that the atria have an opportunity to fully contract before the ventricles signal is permitted to pass down through the ventricles.

The impulse spreads into the ventricles, causing the muscle to contract and to pump out the blood.

The blood from the right ventricle goes to the lungs and the blood from the left ventricle goes to the body.

Pumps in the outside world operate by a rotary mechanism and consume energy to perform mechanical work by moving the fluid. The energy sources vary, including manual operation, electricity, engines, or wind power. However, all are based in principle on the pattern of the original pump, the heart.

Mechanical pumps in the outside world serve in a wide range of applications such as pumping water from wells, aquarium filtering, pond filtering and aeration, in the car industry for water-cooling and fuel injection, in the energy industry for pumping oil and natural gas or for operating cooling towers. In the medical industry, pumps are used for biochemical processes in developing and manufacturing medicine, and as artificial replacements for body parts, in particular the artificial heart.

Many different types of chemical and bio-mechanical pumps have evolved.

I – INTESTINE/WINE PRESS

HUMAN GASTROINTESTINAL TRACT

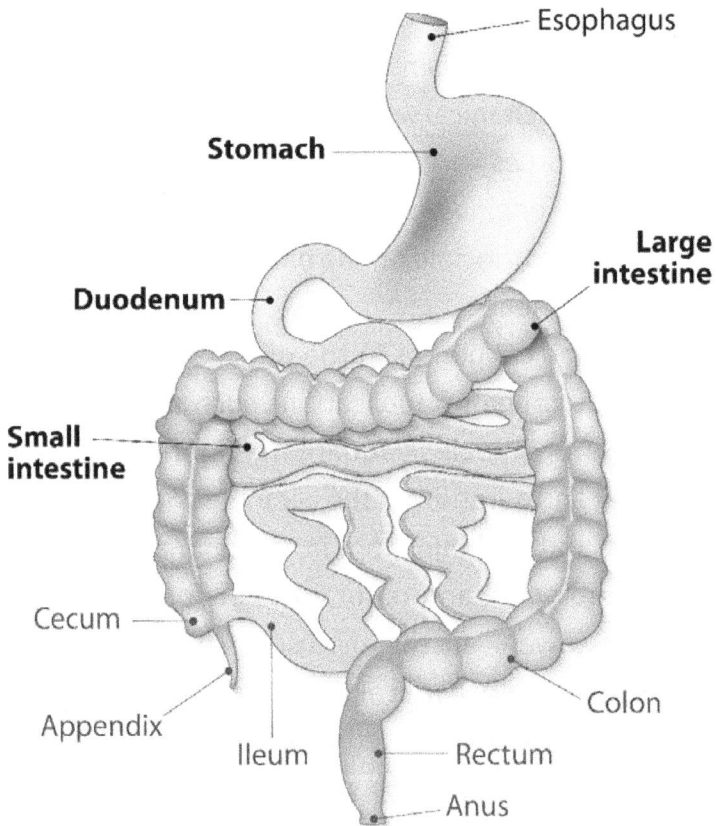

Esophagus

Stomach

Large intestine

Duodenum

Small intestine

Cecum

Appendix

Ileum

Colon

Rectum

Anus

For maintaining a healthy intestine eat a balanced diet, get daily exercise and drink plenty of fluids. You will also prevent digestive distress by getting a good night's sleep and eliminating stress. Consuming enough fibre and avoiding a high-fat diet will also help ensure your small intestine stays in optimal condition.

The small intestine, or small bowel, is a hollow tube about 20 feet long that runs from the stomach to the beginning of the large intestine. The small intestine breaks down food from the stomach and absorbs much of the nutrients from the food and discards the waste.

The small intestine has three parts:

Duodenum

The duodenum is the first part of the small intestine. The main role of the duodenum is to complete the first phase of digestion. In this section of the intestine, food from the stomach is mixed with enzymes from the pancreas and bile from the gallbladder. The enzymes and bile help to break down the food.

Jejunum

The jejunum is the second part of the small intestine. After food is broken down in the duodenum, it moves to the jejunum, where the inside walls absorb the food's nutrients. The inside walls of the jejunum have many circular folds, which make its surface area large enough to absorb all of the nutrients that the body needs.

Ileum

The ileum is the third part of the small intestine. It absorbs bile acids, which are returned to the liver to be made into more bile, then stored in the gallbladder for future use in the duodenum. The ileum also absorbs vitamin B12, which the body uses to make nerve cells and red blood cells.

After food is processed in the small intestine, it passes into the large intestine, also called the large bowel or colon. The large intestine, which is about 5 feet long, extracts most of the water from this food and distributes it to the body; the remaining material passes through the colon and out of the body as faeces.

Like the intestine, the wine press is designed to separate the juice, and nutrients from the pulp / waste. A wine press is a device used to extract juice from crushed grapes during wine making. There are a number of different style of presses that are used by wine makers but their overall function is the same. Each style of press exerts controlled pressure in order to free the juice from the fruit. The most common fruits are grapes.

J –JOINTS /HINGE JOINTS

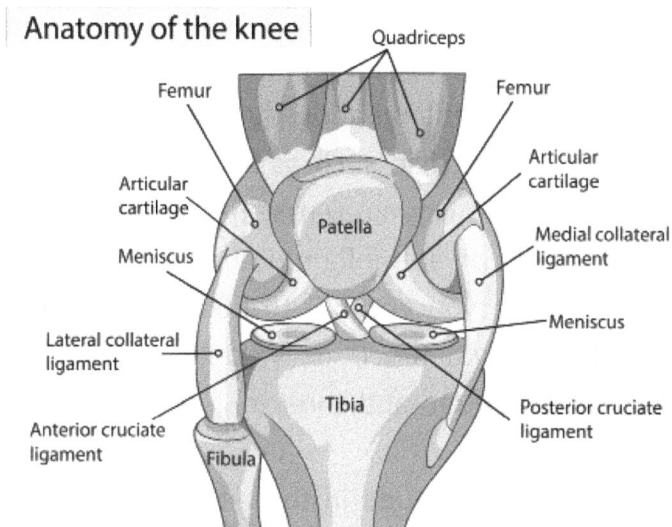

Anatomy of the knee

Quadriceps

Femur

Femur

Articular
cartilage

Articular
cartilage

Patella

Meniscus

Medial collateral
ligament

Lateral collateral
ligament

Meniscus

Tibia

Posterior cruciate
ligament

Anterior cruciate
ligament

Fibula

To keep healthy joints we need to maintain a healthy weight. We must vary our exercise. Working out helps reduce stiffness in the joints. We must not overtax any one area, because that will increase pain. Weight training helps strengthen the muscles and ligaments surrounding joints, protecting them from damage. Modify muscle-building moves so they don't strain the joint of the part you are exercising. People with arthritis can do seated leg lifts instead of squats and lunges, which can increase pressure on the knee. Sit on a chair with both feet on the floor. Bend your knee and raise your leg so it's parallel to the floor. You can do one leg at a time or both.

Eat beneficial foods. Studies show the Omega-3 fatty acids found in fish can help not only reduce symptoms associated with joint pain but also change the levels of inflammation that may be causing some of the pain. Fish oil slows the production of inflammation-signalling cells. The best sources are fish such as salmon and tuna. Research shows vitamin D may help protect your joints, too, via an anti-inflammatory effect.

Make sure you get 400 to 800 International Units (IU) of vitamin D daily; one cup of milk contains 100 (IUs), and three ounces of salmon has 300-650.

Hinge joint is found in the elbow, finger and knee. The elbow joint is the site where the long bone at the top of your arm (the humerus) meets the two bones of your forearm (the radius and the ulna). It's a hinge joint, which means that you can bend your arm in one direction only.

The door hinge attaches the door to the door frame. It keeps the door in place. It functions in a similar way to the joint in the body enabling the door to be opened in one direction only.

K – KIDNEYS/FILTRATION SYSTEM

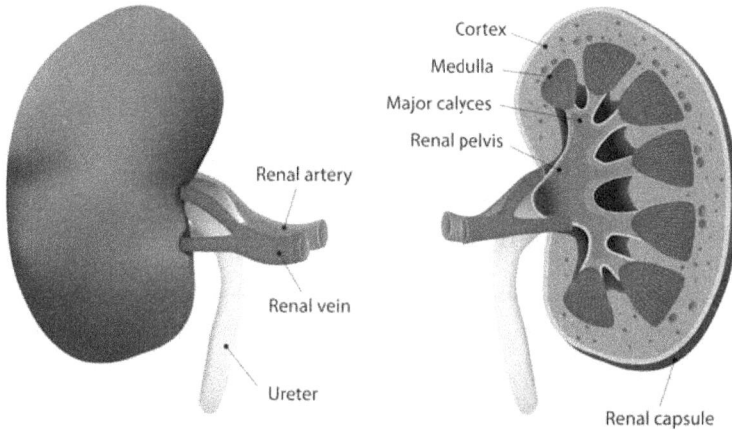

Cortex
Medulla
Major calyces
Renal pelvis
Renal artery
Renal vein
Ureter
Renal capsule

The purpose of your kidneys is to remove waste from your bloodstream (among other functions like producing urine).Water is an important component for all bodily functions, so it's a good idea to make a habit of having a glass of water when you can, at least eight glasses daily. Increase your water intake on particularly hot days or when you are more active than usual. Add a pinch of celtic salt to replace electrolytes.

Every day, the two kidneys filter about 120 to 150 quarts of blood to produce about 1 to 2 quarts of urine, composed of wastes and extra fluid. The urine flows from the kidneys to the bladder through two thin tubes of muscle called ureters, one on each side of the bladder. The bladder stores urine.

In the nephron, (the body of the kidney) approximately 20 percent of the blood gets filtered under pressure through the walls of the glomerular capillaries and Bowman's capsule. The filtrate is composed of water, ions (sodium, potassium, chloride), glucose and small proteins . The rate of filtration is approximately 125 ml/min or 45 gallons (180 litres) each day. Considering that you have 7 to 8 litres of blood in your body, this means that your entire blood volume gets filtered approximately 20 to 25 times each day! Also, the amount of any substance that gets filtered is the product of the concentration of that substance in the blood and the rate of filtration.

So the higher the concentration, the greater the amount filtered or the greater the filtration rate, the more substance gets filtered. The arrangement of the glomerular capillaries in series with the peritubular capillaries is important to maintain a constant pressure in the glomerular capillaries, and thus a constant rate of filtration, despite momentary fluctuations in blood pressure. Once the filtrate has entered the Bowman's capsule, it flows through the lumen of the nephron into the proximal. This filtration system in a coffee machine operates like the kidney in making espresso or cappuccino. In a cappuccino machine, water is forced under pressure through a fine sieve containing ground coffee. The filtrate is the brewed coffee. The sewage disposal uses the same principle of filtration where it removes the debris and waste from the sludge, then the water is purified and recycled.

L –LUNGS (BELLOWS)

ANATOMY OF THE LUNGS

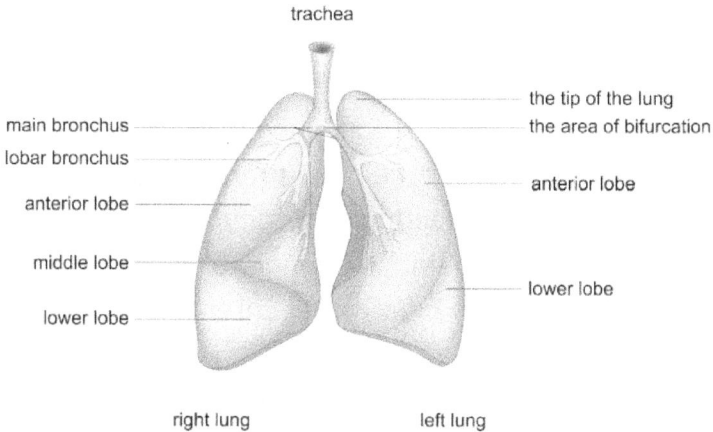

trachea

the tip of the lung
the area of bifurcation

main bronchus

lobar bronchus

anterior lobe

anterior lobe

middle lobe

lower lobe

lower lobe

right lung   left lung

Our lungs need daily care and attention. Breathing feeds oxygen to every cell in the body. Without sufficient oxygen, people are more prone to health problems, including respiratory illnesses, chronic obstructions, pulmonary disease and even heart disease. Everyday breathing isn't enough to keep the oxygen flowing through the body at peak levels. Experts at Rush University Medical Center say, "Lungs at rest and during most daily activities are only at 50 percent of their capacity."

Since regular day-to-day activity doesn't help

you use your lungs to full capacity, you need to challenge the lungs with more intense activity. "And to help counteract the build-up of toxins and tar in the lungs caused by environmental pollutants, allergens, dust and cigarette smoke, you need to help your lungs cleanse themselves," Diaphragmatic breathing uses the awareness of the diaphragm muscle, which separates the organs in the abdomen from the lungs."By concentrating on lowering the diaphragm as you breathe in, you'll get a much deeper inhale," says Roberts. "This is the technique that professional singers use to increase their lung capacity."

The lungs' main function is to help oxygen from the air we breathe to enter the red cells in the blood. Red blood cells, also known as eurothocytes then carry oxygen around the body to be used in the cells found in our body for oxidation which is commonly known as burning. This process releases energy from chemical bonds of the food we eat.

The Bellows are used to blow air over lighted coal or wood to provide oxygen to cause the substance to burn, releasing energy from the burning material.

The term "bellows" is used by extension for a flexible bag whose volume can be changed by compression or expansion.

A bellows or pair of bellows is a device constructed to furnish a strong blast of air. The simplest type consists of a flexible bag comprising a pair of rigid boards with handles joined by flexible leather sides enclosing an approximately airtight cavity which can be expanded and contracted by operating the handle. This device is fitted with a valve allowing air to fill the cavity when expanded, and with a tube through which the air is forced out in a stream when the cavity is compressed. It has many applications, in particular blowing on a fire to supply it with air.

MITOCHONDRION/ ELECTRICAL GENERATOR

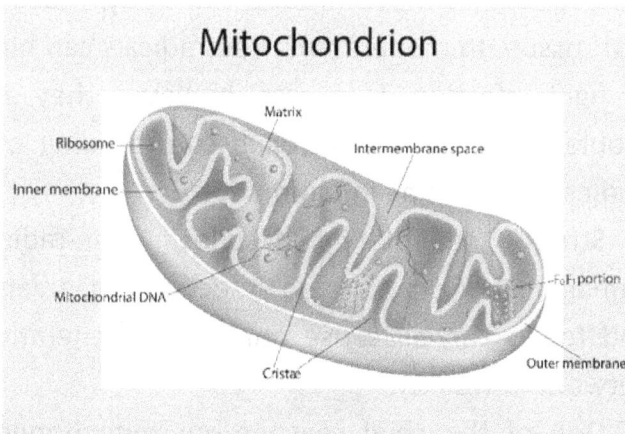

Mitochondrion

Matrix
Ribosome
Intermembrane space
Inner membrane
Mitochondrial DNA
F$_0$F$_1$ portion
Cristae
Outer membrane

Mitochondrion is an organelle found inside cells which produces energy by breaking down food. It releases that energy along with some by products, carbon dioxide, and free radicals.

Each mitochondrion is filled with some 17,000

biochemical assembly lines, all designed to produce a molecule called adenosine triphosphate, or ATP.

The more energy a tissue or organ demands for proper function, the more mitochondria its cells contain. Mitochondria are especially abundant in the cells that make up our hearts, brains, and muscles.

The density and health of the mitochondria in your organs and muscles are, a reflection of your current level of health and fitness. (Lean muscle tissue, for example, contains far more mitochondria than fat.)

Free radicals are charged, highly active molecules that move around the body, reacting with tissue. In moderation, free radicals can help us fight infection. In excess, however, they are problematic, damaging cell tissue, eroding our bodies, and causing inflammation.

Stress, sedentary lifestyles, free-radical damage, and exposure to infections, allergens, and toxins can all cause our energy-generation network to weaken.

One of the chief reasons our mitochondria deteriorate, says Cohen, is that we eat an excess of poor-quality foods and a deficit of healthy ones. Mitochondrias are well-defined cytoplasmic organelles of the cell which take part in a variety of cellular metabolic functions. Survival of the cells requires energy to perform different functions. The mitochondria are important as these organelles supply all the necessary biological energy of the cells, and they obtain this energy by oxidizing the substrates of the Krebs cycle.

The main function of the Krebs cycle is energy production, The Krebs cycle, also known as the tricarboxylic acid cycle or the citric acid cycle, is at the centre of cellular metabolism.

There are eight reactions in the Krebs cycle. The Krebs cycle finishes the breakdown of sugar and produces adenosine triphosphate, called ATP. ATP is the molecular currency of the cells and stores and transports energy within it. The Krebs cycle also provides electrons for the process of oxidative phosphorylation. Oxidative phosphorylation is a major source of ATP and energy. The Krebs cycle takes place in the mitochondria. Hence, the mitochondria referred to as the 'power of the cell'. Almost all the eukaryotic cells or red blood cells have mitochondria.

The Mitochondria, in the human body, is a device that converts mechanical energy obtained from an external source into electrical energy output. The generator uses mechanical energy supplied to force the movement of electric charges present in the wire of its windings through an external electric circuit. It is similar to a water pump which causes the flow of water running through it. The modern-day generator works on the principle of electromagnetic induction discovered by Michael Faraday in 1831-32. Faraday discovered that the above flow of electric charges could be induced by moving an electrical conductor, such as a wire that contains electric charges, in a magnetic field. This movement creates a voltage difference between the two ends of the wire or electrical conductor, which in turn causes the electric charges to flow, thus generating electric current.

N- NERVOUS SYSTEM /
PHONE SYSTEM

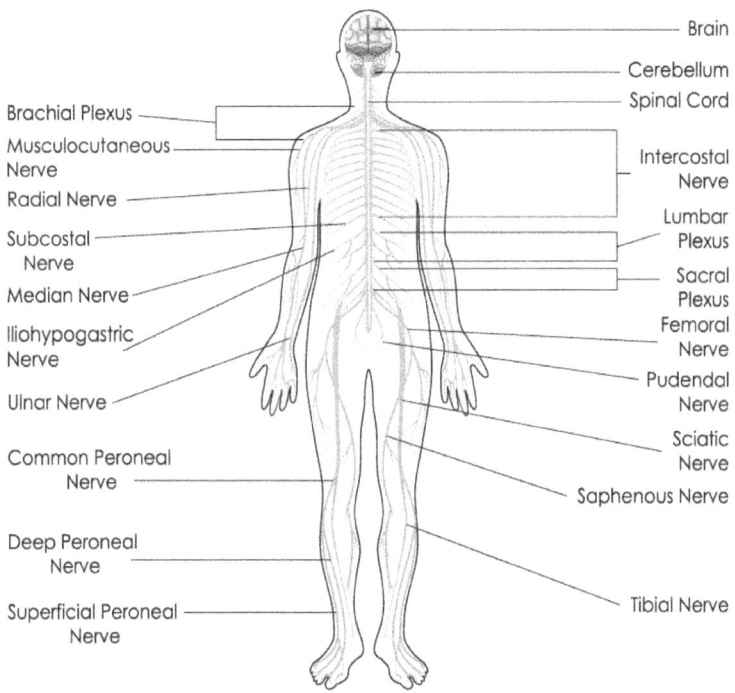

Brachial Plexus

Musculocutaneous
Nerve

Radial Nerve

Subcostal
Nerve

Median Nerve

Iliohypogastric
Nerve

Ulnar Nerve

Common Peroneal
Nerve

Deep Peroneal
Nerve

Superficial Peroneal
Nerve

Brain

Cerebellum

Spinal Cord

Intercostal
Nerve

Lumbar
Plexus

Sacral
Plexus

Femoral
Nerve

Pudendal
Nerve

Sciatic
Nerve

Saphenous Nerve

Tibial Nerve

The human nervous system represents a vast network of receptors that continually sense and respond to both internal and external stimuli. Nutritional deficiencies negatively affect your nervous system, They can cause nerve damage and lead to a range of symptoms. Foods especially rich in brain-friendly nutrients help your nervous system function at an optimal level.

Vitamin B-1 or thiamine plays an essential

role in the maintenance of nerve health. The diet include Brewer's yeast, beef liver, eggs, seafood, sunflower seeds and beans. The nervous system requires vitamin B-6 to produce serotonin and two important neurotransmitters involved in nerve cell communication. Healthy dopamine levels play a role in the reward system in your brain, the region that affects how your body reacts to food, as well as other compounds while serotonin promotes mental health. Good dietary sources of vitamin B6 include potatoes, bananas, fortified cereals and chick peas.

Vitamin B-12 deficiency harms the nervous system and can cause symptoms such as numbness and tingling in the feet and hands. Sources of vitamin B-12, are fish, meat, eggs and dairy products.

Copper helps to produce neurotransmitters, making it essential for brain function. If you become severely deficient in copper certain serious neuro-logical conditions may occur, including copper deficiency myelopathy, a progressive loss of nerve function caused by degeneration of the spinal cord. Sources of copper include prunes, dark leafy green vegetables such as kale and spinach, small oysters, shell fish and nuts.

The nervous system is a complex network of interconnected excitable cells. These cells, called neurons, are capable of transmitting an electrochemical signal when appropriately stimulated. Normally, a slight negative electrical potential is maintained in the neurons (relative to the outside) and this is momentarily reversed during transmission of nerve impulse.

Activation of neuron cell and generation of a nerve impulse that moves forward from its point of origin is known as action potential. As already mentioned, the inside of a neuron is slightly electrically negative. The nerve impulses are propagated in the form of this electrical activity caused by an action potential.

The telephone is connected through wires caring electoral impulse. When the caller lifts the handset and dials the central processing unit identifies the calling line and sends the dialling tone to the requesting party like the brain when it receives the message. The caller then dials the desired number. During this time, the number dialled is succesfully received, analysed and transferred to the controller. If the line is busy, the caller hears the engaged tone.

Like the nervous system it uses an all or nothing rule, messages transfer electrically once stimulated.

When the person being called picks up the phone, the connection is established in the same way when the organ receives the stimulation a connection is made, if the organ is not functioning properly e.g diseased, no connection is made;

Disconnection occurs when one of the two speakers hangs up again.

O –OESOPHAGUS/
NON RETURNABLE VALVE

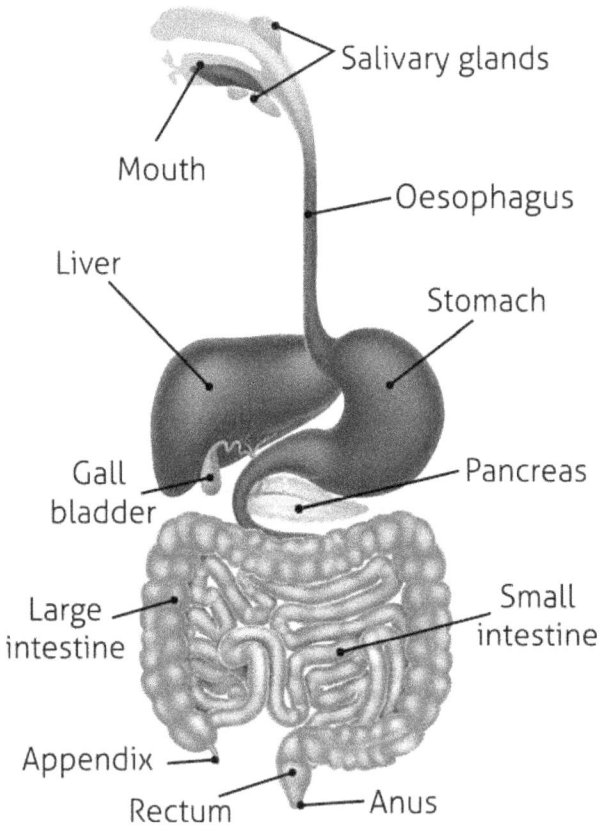

Salivary glands

Mouth

Oesophagus

Liver

Stomach

Gall bladder

Pancreas

Large intestine

Small intestine

Appendix

Rectum

Anus

To maintain a healthy oesophagus or gullet all fruits and vegetables especially kale and broccoli are beneficial, whole wheat grains protect against esophageal cancer. Whole grains such as brown rice, quinoa, oats and whole wheat bread are rich in dietary fiber. Such fibres as kale, cabbage and apricots help foods pass smoothly and efficiently through your body.

The Oesophagus (Gullet) is a tunnel which channels the bulbous mass of food from the mouth to directly pass through the throat into the stomach. It prevents food from escaping into the wind pipe which cause one to choke or in the blood system which would stimulate the immune system to provide defence. This can have an adverse effect as in the development of (MS) Multiple Sclorosis the immune system attack the nervous system causing scarring which is the cause of neurological conditions.

A non-return valve is a mechanical device that normally allows fluid to flow through it in only one direction. The force of upstream fluid creates high differential pressure across the interior valve body, and it then allows forward streams to pass through.

An important concept in valves is the cracking pressure, which is the minimum upstream pressure required for the valve to operate. Typically, the valve is designed for a specific cracking pressure.

the valves are useful in several different types of devices. They stop flooding in water-related devices such as sump pumps and water heaters. They also protect equipment that can be harmed by the reverse flow of material, such as control valves, strainers and flow meters. In addition, the valves can stop material from constantly flowing backwards when a device is off, which can save power and protect the parts of the device.This is a pipe which allows water to flow in one direction.

The Oesophagus prevents the food from getting into the wrong parts of the blood system which could foster neurological damage. The tunnel protects people and things.

P- PENIS/ RUBBER TUBING

It is important to maintain personal hygiene of the penis, but excessive washing with soap and detergents can make you sore. You should wash your penis gently and retract the foreskin regularly (such as when you have a bath or shower). Check your testicles this is to detect any changes in the scrotum at the earliest possible stage. It is essential that young men should be aware of any lump in the testes.

Corpus cavernossum are two columns of tissue running along the sides of the penis. Blood fills this tissue to cause an erection.

Corpus spongiosum is a column of sponge-like tissue that surrounds the urethra in the penis and ends at the glans penis; it fills with blood during an erection, keeping the urethra - which runs through it - open.

The urethra runs through the corpus spongiosum, conducting urine out of the body. An erection results from changes in blood flow in the penis. When a man becomes sexually aroused, nerves cause the penis blood vessels to expand. More blood flows in and less flows out of the penis, hardening the tissue in the corpus cavernosum.

Air-filled tyres are a requirement for a comfortable ride, but keeping that high-pressure air sealed inside the tyre for extended periods of time is a challenge. Using a tube separates the air-sealing functionality from the structural and wear-resisting functionality of the rim, spokes, and tyre, which makes it easier to design and manufacture. Tubeless tires have more stringent requirements on the rim and the tyre bead to seal properly.

Rubber tubing is used in tyres. When air is pulled into it becomes taut.

Q – QUADRICEPS FEMORIS/ TRAIN WHEEL

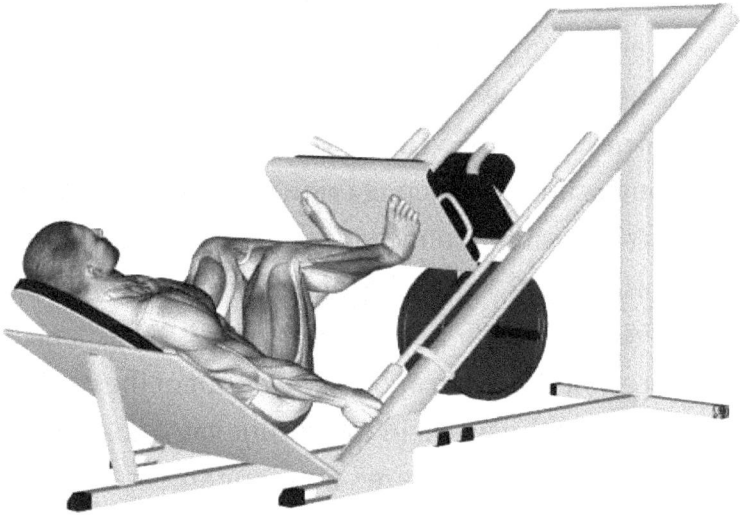

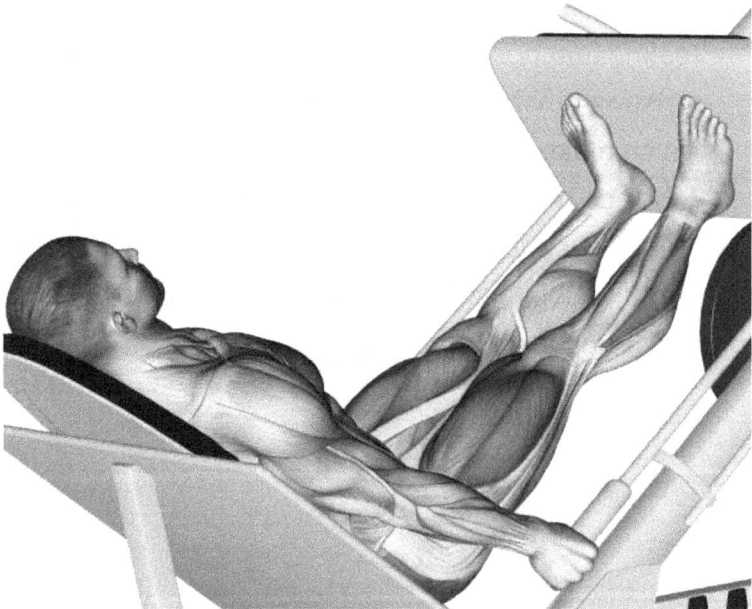

The quadriceps femoris is a large extensor muscle of the anterior thigh, composed of the rectus femoris, the vastus lateralis, the vastus medialis, and the vastus intermedius. The quadriceps forms a large dense mass covering the front and sides of the femur. Tendons of the four parts of the muscle unite at the distal part of the thigh, forming a single strong tendon that embeds the patella and inserts onto the tibial tuberosity. The muscle functions to extend the leg.

This muscle connects the knee joint and hip joint it enables the two joints to work together yet it does not just stabilises the two body parts.

Exercise is a simple way to get your quad muscles working properly.

• Lie on your back on a flat surface.

• Bend the knee of your uninvolved leg (the one that is stationary) to a 90-degree angle, and keep your foot flat on the surface. Keep your in-volved leg straight without the knee bent.

• Slowly lift the involved leg 12 inches off the floor (by contracting the front thigh muscles). Hold for five seconds.

• Slowly lower your leg to the floor. Relax and repeat 10 to 15 times.

The knee of the raised leg should remain straight throughout this exercise. Focus on lifting by using the muscles on the front of your hip joint. This exercise can be made more challenging by placing a 2 or 3-pound cuff weight on your ankle before you lift. Repeat exercise with the other leg.

There are two parallel pieces of metals that keep two small wheels together to be able to sit stable on the train track. Like the muscles, the bars don't bend or move but they enable the wheels to move together.

R -RIB CAGE/CAGE

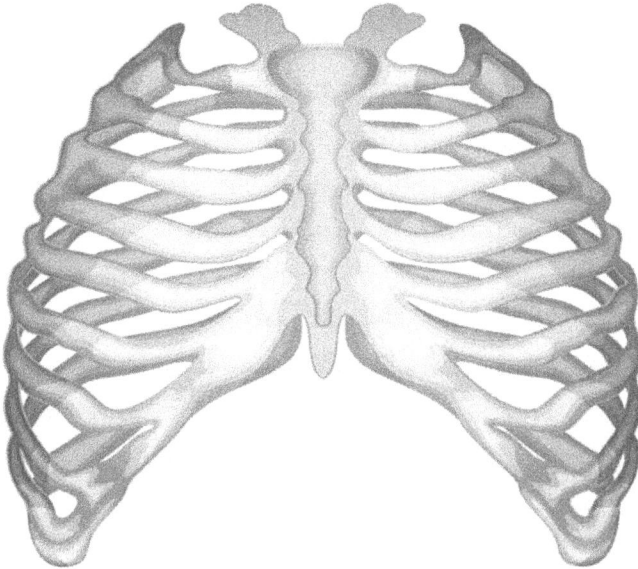

This is formed by the vertebral column, ribs and sternum and encloses the heart and lungs. In humans, the rib cage, also known as the thoracic cage, is a bony and cartilaginous structure which surrounds the thoracic cavity and supports the pectoral girdle (shoulder girdle), forming a core portion of the human skeleton. The rib cage protects vital organs, such as the heart and lungs. Three types of bones form one's rib cage: the sternum, ribs and thoracic vertebra protect the vital organs of the chest cavity (the heart, lungs and major blood vessels), and support the shoulder girdle and upper extremities and provide the anchors of many muscles of the neck, back, chest and shoulders. Finally the intercostal space (between ribs) is occupied by the intercostal muscles that lift and depress the chest during breathing.

Like the rib cage, a metal cage is built to protect things from getting in or out except by the person in charge of the cage, for example, around a house to keep out intruders, around electric generators or appliances to prevent them from being stolen.

SKELETON/BUILDING FRAME

The skeletal system provides support and structure to the body and serves to protect vital organs, such as your brain, heart and lungs. Working with muscles, the skeletal system assists in movement. While bones are hard, they can be broken and weakened if not cared for properly. A good diet and regular exercise will help keep your skeletal system strong and healthy.

Eat calcium-rich foods. This is especially true for people over age 40, when natural bone replacement slows down. Milk, cheese and other dairy products contain calcium. Broccoli, kale, sardines, salmon, Brazil nuts, almonds, oranges and calcium-fortified foods are good sources of calcium as well.

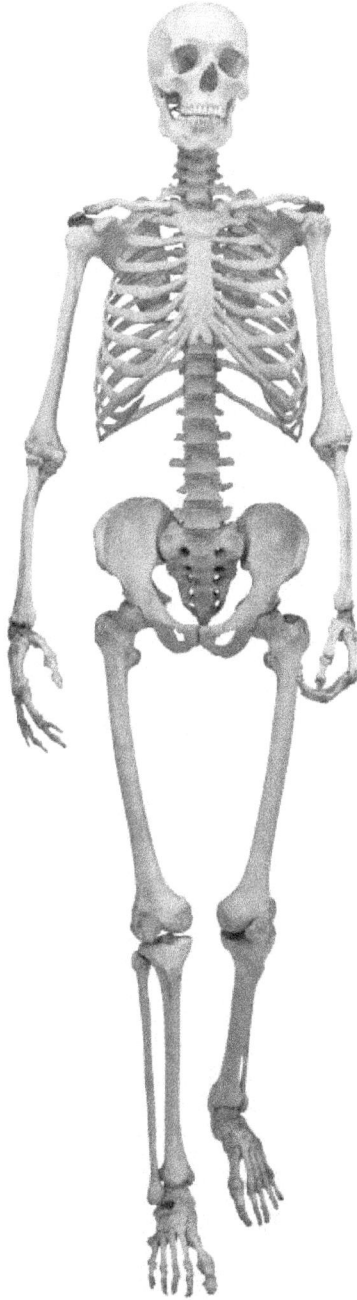

The American Academy of Orthopedic Surgeons indi-cates that getting 1,000 mg of calcium through diet alone may be difficult and therefore suggests a vitamin supplement as well.

Eat foods with vitamin D to assist in calcium absorption. Adults need 15 mg of vitamin D a day. Foods with vitamin D include dairy, eggs, fatty fish such as salmon or tuna and fortified orange juice and cereal. Exposure to the sun triggers vitamin D synthesis to produce vitamin D as well.

Perform at least 30 minutes of weight-bearing exercise at least twice a week. Building muscle increases bone density to build healthy bones and prevent osteoporosis. Push-ups, squats and planks strengthen muscles over most of the body. As you get stronger, using dumbbells increases the resistance to maintain your strength.

Avoid smoking and drinking. The Mayo Clinic.com reports that tobacco use and consuming more than two alcoholic drinks a day may contribute to weak bones and osteoporosis.

Discuss potential side effects of medication with your doctor. Some medicines can weaken bones and increase your risk of osteoporosis. Your doctor will be able to prescribe bone-boosting medication if needed.

Protect the body. Wear your seat belt when driving and a helmet when using a motorcycle. Use headgear when engaged in sports that could lead to brain damage such as rugby, skating.

The skeletal system in the body provides shape, supports and protects organs and the soft areas of the body. Its other functions are bodily movement, producing blood for the body and storing minerals that the physical structure needs. It shapes and supports.

The skeleton is made up of various bones and provides the framework for the body.

Like the skeletal structure of the body, the building frame provides shape, structure and support to a building. It is the fitting together of framing materials, which are usually wood, engineered wood, or structural steel. Building framing is divided into two broad categories, heavy-frame construction (heavy framing) and smaller called light-frame construction. Use of minimal structural material allows builders to enclose a large area with minimal cost, while achieving a wide variety of architectural styles. Historically mankind fitted naturally shaped wooden poles together as framework and then began using joints to connect the timbers, a method today called traditional timber framing.

Modern light-frame structures usually gain strength from rigid panels (plywood and other plywood-like composites such as oriented strand board (OSB) used to form all or part of wall sections) but recently carpenters employed various forms of diagonal bracing to stabilize walls. Diagonal bracing remains a vital interior part of many roof systems.

T- TEETH / KNIVES

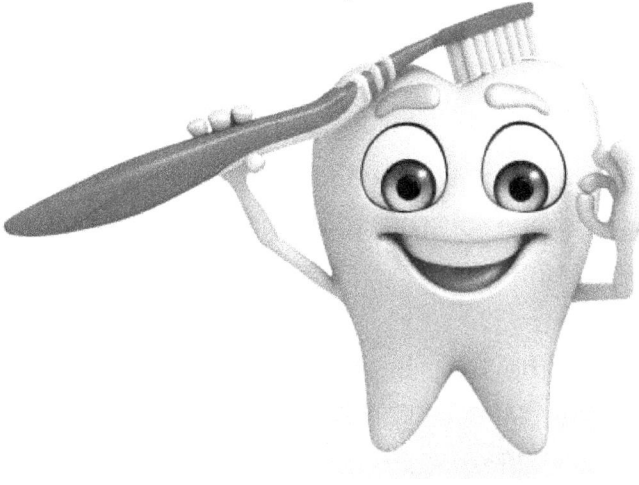

There are five basic steps to caring for the human teeth and gums:

1. Brushing
2. Flossing
3. Rinsing
4. Eating right
5. Visiting the dentist

Brush them optimally twice a day, brush after every meal. Ideally wait 30 minutes after eating, this will allow any enamel that might have softened from acid during eating to re-harden and not get brushed away. Brushing removes plaque, a film of bacteria that clings to teeth.

When bacteria in plaque comes into contact with food, they produce acids. These acids lead to cavities. To brush:

• Place a pea-sized dab of fluoride toothpaste on the head of the tooth-brush. (Use a soft toothbrush.)

• Place the toothbrush against the teeth at a 45-degree angle up to the mouth
There are different kinds of teeth, Teeth help you chew your food, making it easier to digest. Each type of tooth has a slightly different shape and performs a different job. Types of teeth include:

• Incisors. Incisors are the eight teeth in the front and centre of your mouth (four on top and four on bottom). These are the teeth that you use to take bites of your food. Incisors are usually the first teeth to erupt at around 6 months of age for your first set of teeth, and between 6 and 8 years of age for your adult set.

• Canines. Your four canines are the next type of teeth to develop. These are your sharpest teeth and are used for ripping and tearing food apart. Primary canines generally appear between 16 and 20 months of age with the upper canines coming in just ahead of the lower canines. In permanent teeth, the order is reversed. Lower canines erupt around age 9 with the uppers arriving between 11 and 12 years of age.

Premolars. Premolars, or bicuspids, are used for chewing and grinding food. You have four premolars on each side of your mouth, two on the upper and two on the lower jaw. The first premolars appear around age 10 and the second premolars arrive about a year later.

Molars. Primary molars are also used for chewing and grinding food. These appear between 12 and 15 years of age. These molars, also known as deciduous molars, are replaced by the first and second permanent premolars (four upper and four lower). The permanent molars do not replace, but come in behind the primary teeth. The first molars erupt around 6 years of age (before the primary molars fall out) while the second molars come in between 11 and 13 years of age

Like the teeth, knives are tools for cutting and piercing. Daggers are used primarily for piercing, standard for cutting. The serrated knife is for grinding things. Like the varied shapes in the human teeth, knife blades are similarly designed. The Incisors are pointed teeth and a knife normally has a point which punctures and assists dissecting. Canine teeth are used for cutting the food similarly to a knife used for cutting. The Premolar and Molars are somewhat serrated like a serrated bread knife which deals with the more intricate cutting matters.

U - UMBIBILICAL CORD/
INTER VENOUS CORD

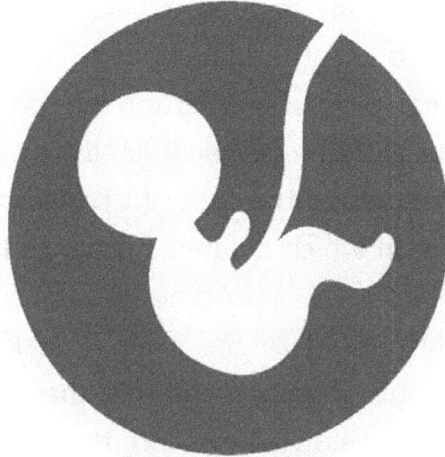

The umbilical cord (also called the birth cord) connects the developing foetus (developing infant in mother's womb) to the placenta (an organ with nutrients in the womb for feeding the developing infant). It functions as a lifeline, connecting the vulnerable foetus to its mother and delivering vital nutrients and oxygen, while carrying away waste materials.

A fully-developed umbilical cord is typically between 18 and 24 inches in length and nearly an inch in diameter. It contains three distinct blood vessels: one vein (that carries oxygenated and nutrient-rich blood to the foetus) and two arteries (that carry depleted blood away from the foetus).

The umbilical cord is coated in a substance called Wharton's jelly, which serves to strengthen the cord and protect the blood vessels inside

This is especially important because the foetus is unable to breathe (having neither functioning lungs nor an oxygen source) and the cord provides the foetus with the oxygen it needs to live.

A continuous intravenous (IV) drip is a medical procedure in which a liquid substance is directly dripped into a vein over time through a tube and needle inserted into the skin. A sealed device called a drip chamber controls the process so the substance slowly flows into the vein, without any chance of air entering the bloodstream. Air introduced into the bloodstream can create serious health problems and can even be fatal.

A continuous intravenous drip, also called an IV drip, functions similarly to the Umbilical Cord. It is a medical device which enables a liquid substance to go directly into a vein. It is commonly associated with long-term treatments, but it is also used as a short-term method to rehydrate patients or give them medicine or nutrients to revitalize them. It's a very efficient process to quickly supply the entire body with prescribed medicine. IV drips are routinely used in hospitals as well as in clinics and doctor's offices that prepare patients for admittance to hospitals.

There are two common types of lines used for intravenous drips. A peripheral intravenous drip line is used to access peripheral veins, or those located anywhere except the abdomen or chest. The other is used in the right atrium of the heart or in areas adjacent to the heart. It is referred to as a central intravenous drip line.

Like the umbilical cord this intravenous cord or tube helps to sustain human life.

V – VERTEBRA/FULCRUM

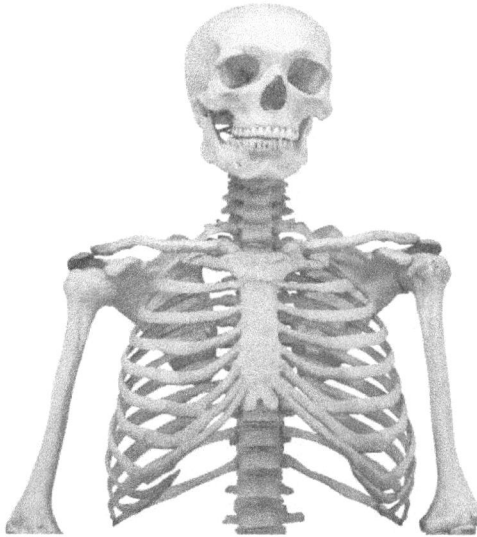

The skeletal system provides support and structure to the body and serves to protect vital organs such as your brain, heart and lungs. Working with muscles, the skeletal system assists in movement. While bones are hard, they can be broken and weakened if not cared for properly.

A good diet and regular exercise will help keep your skeletal system strong and healthy. Eat calcium-rich foods.

This is especially true for people over age 40, when natural bone replacement slows down. Milk, cheese and other dairy products contain calcium. Broccoli, kale, sardines, salmon, Brazil nuts, almonds, oranges and calcium-fortified foods are good sources of calcium as well.

Eat foods with vitamin D to assist in calcium absorption. Foods with vitamin D include dairy, eggs, fatty fish such as salmon or tuna and fortified orange juice and cereal. Exposure to the sun triggers vitamin D synthesis to produce vitamin D, as well.

Perform at least 30 minutes of weight-bearing exercise at least twice a week. Building muscle increases bone density to build healthy bones and prevent osteoporosis.

Avoid smoking and drinking. Discuss potential side effects of medication with your doctor. Some medicines can weaken bones and increase your risk of osteoporosis.

Protect the body. Wear your seat belt when driving and a helmet when using a motorcycle. Use headgear when engaged in sports that could lead to brain damage such as football, in-line skating.

The vertebrae in the human vertebral column are divided into different regions, which correspond to the curves of the spinal column. The articulating vertebrae are named according to their region of the spine. Vertebrae in these regions are essentially alike, with minor variation.

These regions are called the cervical spine, thoracic spine, lumbar spine, sacrum and coccyx. There are seven cervical vertebrae, twelve thoracic vertebrae and five lumbar vertebrae. The number of vertebrae in a region can vary but overall the number remains the same. The number of those in the cervical region however is only rarely changed. The vertebrae of the cervical, thoracic and lumbar spines are independent bones, and generally quite similar. The vertebrae of the sacrum and coccyx are usually fused and unable to move independently. Two special vertebrae are the atlas and axis, on which the head rests. The atlas is the first of the seven cervical vertebrae and bears the direct weight of the skull. The axis is the second of the seven cervical vertebrae; it allows axial (rotational) movement of the skull.

The atlas sits on a pin that sticks up from the axis. This allows the head to move in all directions, from nodding to turning.

A fulcrum, or pivot point, is the area around which a lever turns. A lever is a hard length of material or a bar - used to put out force or maintain weight at one end, while pressure is exerted on its second end. In other words, when force is placed on one end of a bar or handle, which turns on the third point, or fulcrum, force or weight, is managed on the second point of the lever.

A good example of a lever and its accompanying pivot point is a child's see-saw. The ends of the see-saw, where participants sit, would be considered points one and two. The fulcrum is the area in the middle upon which the lever balances. When one participant pushes his or her weight, the pivot point in the center supports the motion of the second point on the lever either raising or lowering.

For the example of the see-saw, a class one lever, the weight is more or less distributed evenly by the pivot point because it is generally placed in the middle of the lever. In other words, the fulcrum is in between the force applied to one end, or input effort, and the resulting force, or output load. However, this is not always the case in lever and fulcrum relationships.

W - WOMB/INCUBATOR

The uterus, also commonly known as the womb, is a hollow muscular organ of the female reproductive system that is responsible for housing the embryo and foetus during pregnancy. An incredibly distensible organ, the uterus can expand during pregnancy from around the size of a closed fist to become large enough to hold a full term baby. It is also an incredibly strong organ, able to contract forcefully.

The uterus has the ability to nurture the fertilized ovum that develops into the foetus and to hold it till the baby is mature enough for birth. The fertilized ovum gets implanted into the endometrium and derives nourishment from blood vessels which develop exclusively for this purpose.

In biology, an incubator is a device used to grow and maintain microbiological cultures or cell culture and end foetuses also used to care for immature foetuses. The incubator maintains optimal temperature, humidity and other conditions such as the carbon dioxide and oxygen content of the atmosphere inside.

X & Y CHROMOSOMES/ZIP

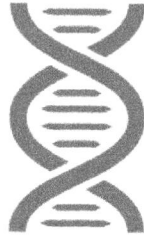

The X and Y chromosomes are the two sex-determining chromosomes and are not found in both males and females. The X chromosome determines the female gender, this happens when X chromosome from the mother lines up and matches like the teeth of a zip with X chromosome from father and the male gender when Y chromosome from father zips up with a the X chromosome from the mother.

A chromosome is a DNA molecule (a group of atoms forming a unit) with part or all of the genetic material of an organism. Chromosomes are normally visible under a light microscope only when the cell is undergoing the metaphase of cell division. Before this happens, every chromosome is copied once, and the copy is joined to the original by a centromere (a central point where two chromosomes tie together), resulting in an X-shaped structure.

As the two chromosomes align themselves to become one structure so the teeth of the two sides of the zipper interlock to become one structure.

The zipper/ fastener is one of the simplest machines of modern times and arguably one of the least essential, but it is an useful device in our everyday lives. It makes it easier to close a pants fly, a suitcase, the back of a dress, a sleeping bag or a tent flap with a zipper than with buttons or cords.

In this article, we'll examine the various parts that make up a zipper and see how these components lock together so easily and securely. The system is ingenious in its simplicity.

SLIDER

The slider joins or separates the elements when the zipper is opened or closed. Various types of sliders are available depending on use.

ELEMENTS

The teeth, also known as elements, are the parts on each side of a zipper that mesh, or engage, with each other when passed through the slider. When the left and the right side teeth are en-gaged they are called chain.

TAPE

The tape is manufactured exclusively for zippers. It is usually made of polyester, but depend-ing on use, synthetic fibre tape, vinyl tape and cotton tape are also available

ZYGOTE/ALLOY
(Genetics)

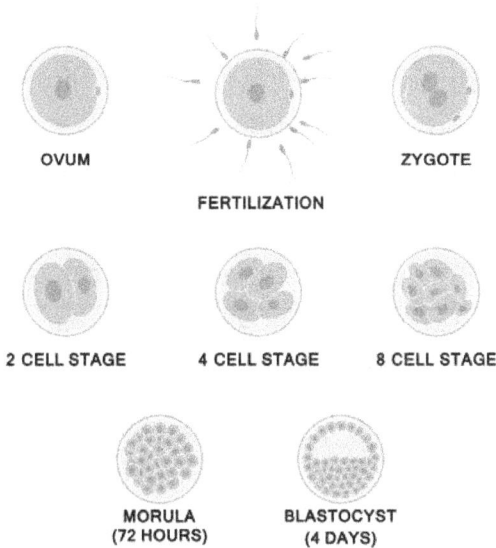

OVUM

FERTILIZATION

ZYGOTE

2 CELL STAGE

4 CELL STAGE

8 CELL STAGE

MORULA
(72 HOURS)

BLASTOCYST
(4 DAYS)

A zygote is a diploid cell (two sets of molecules matching and joined together like when the teeth of the zip joined together resulting from the union of one structure. Half is from the male, it is known as a haploid spermatozoon and half from female ovum (including the organism that develops from that cell). Fertilized ovum organism, being-a living thing that has (or can develop) the ability to act or function independently.

An Alloy is a metal that is formed when two metals combine together. The new metal formed often enhances its properties. For example, the combination of carbon with iron produces steel, which is stronger than iron, its primary element. The electrical and thermal conductivity of alloys is usually lower than that of the pure metals. The physical properties, such as density, reactivity, of an alloy may not differ greatly from those of its base element, but engineering properties such as tensile strength, ductility, and shear strength may be substantially different from those of the constituent materials. This is sometimes a result of the sizes of the atoms in the alloy, because larger atoms exert a compressive force on neighbouring atoms, and smaller atoms exert a tensile force on their neighbours, helping the alloy resist deformation. Sometimes alloys may exhibit marked differences in behaviour even when small amounts of one element are present.

Conclusion

I truly believe our body is the template of every system, machine and organisation that has been or will ever be in existence.

Finally, I believe that the car in some ways is similar to the human body. The engine is like the brain, the exhaust expels waste material like the urethra and the skin. The chassis is similar to the skeletal system of the body because it supports and provides attachment for parts of the car.

Like the body, the car requires food (petrol) and air for oxygen to produce energy.

In the same way that we need to take our car in for a service to keep it running smoothly, so too do we need to look after our bodies to keep them healthy. We need to both look after those things that are without as well as those that are within.

By being aware of our amazing body, and knowing how to look after it well, it will last us a lifetime!

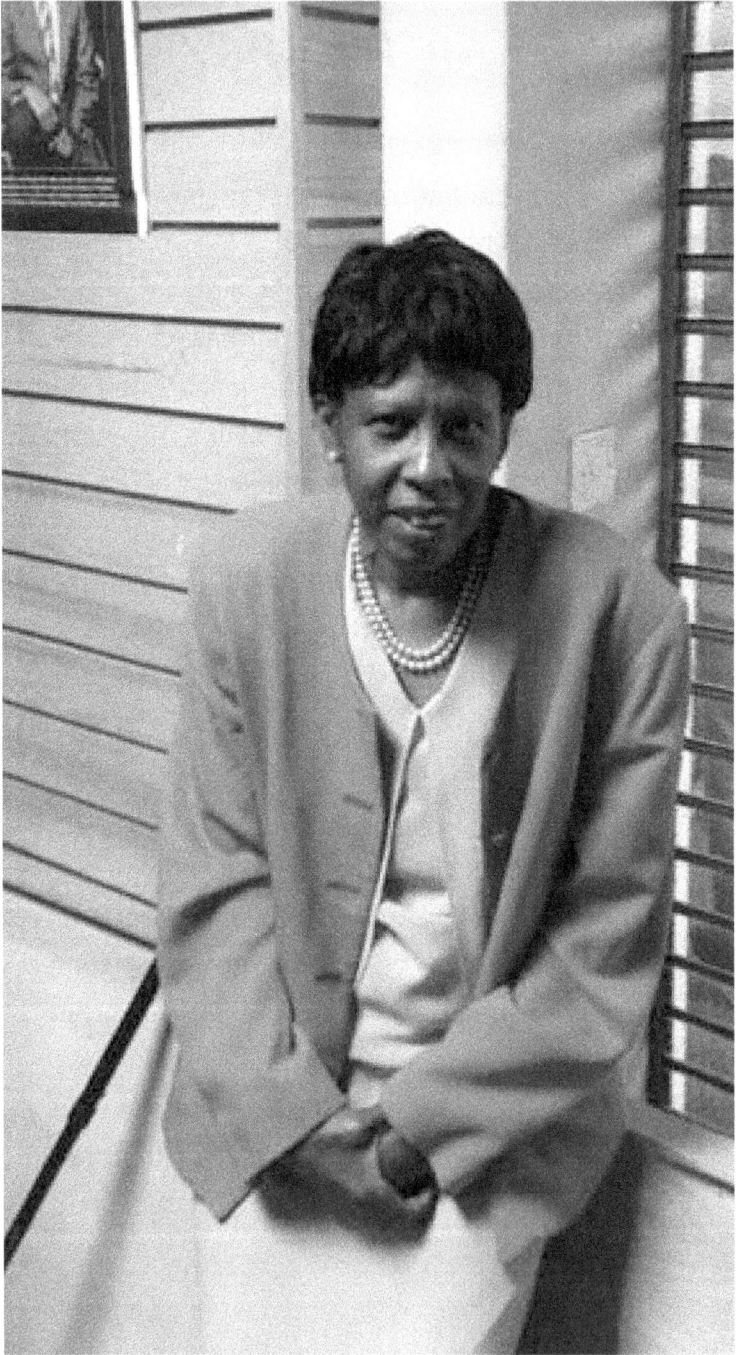

About the Author

Karlene Rickard is a childcare expert who has overcome paralysis in order to write an acclaimed parent's guide to raising happy, well-adjusted children.

Karlene began her career as a science teacher and later got involved in community work and counselling. She has worked extensively as a parent facilitator, trainer and counsellor in the UK, USA, Jamaica, Grenada and Trinidad for over fifteen years. Her powerful 'Empowerment for Parents' parenting programme is credited with changing lives and creating happier families.

She co-founded KJ Academy, a supplementary school in Leyton, East London, and a nursery/infant school in Jamaica where she worked holistically with families to develop their confidence and self-worth.

Karlene is determined to do all she can to have a positive and lasting impact on society through empowering families to raise their children as happy, successful adults who will build healthy communities.

She created the 'Empowerment for Parents' programme and published The A to Z of Parenting, a simple, easy-to-digest guide. Unlike other childcare manuals, the guide places equal emphasis on the well-being of both parent and child, recognising that physically and emotionally stressed adults are unlikely to be great parents, in spite of their best intentions.

Karlene was one of the pioneer facilitators in the UK of the innovative programme Strengthening Families, Strengthening Communities, and she presented the programme in the USA at a fatherhood conference in 2001.

Karlene's book The A to Z of Parenting deals with parents giving clear and honest feedback to their children and dealing with behavioural challenges. It highlights the value of spending quality time with children, outlines ways to educate them in the early years and focuses on the critical life skills that will carry them through to successful adulthood.

Karlene was awarded the Millennium Award in 1999 for developing a parenting programme for African Caribbean families.

Karlene's autobiography *He Speaks* has been widely read and has spread her message that positive relationship, genuine love and being attuned to the voice of God is essential to building well-balanced adults. She has achieved all of this despite the challenge of living with Multiple Sclerosis.

Mary Crowley OBE
Chair, International Federation for Parenting Education

www.ingramcontent.com/pod-product-compliance
Lightning Source LLC
Chambersburg PA
CBHW060346050426
42336CB00050B/2149